SUPER
MATTHEW

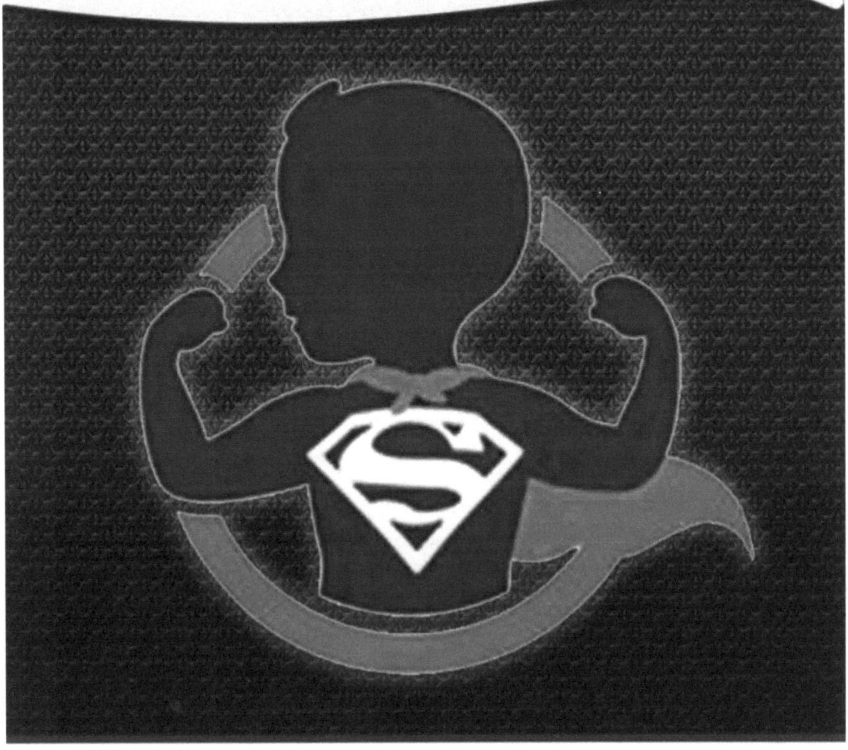

TEAM MATTHEW

Super Matthew

by Team Matthew

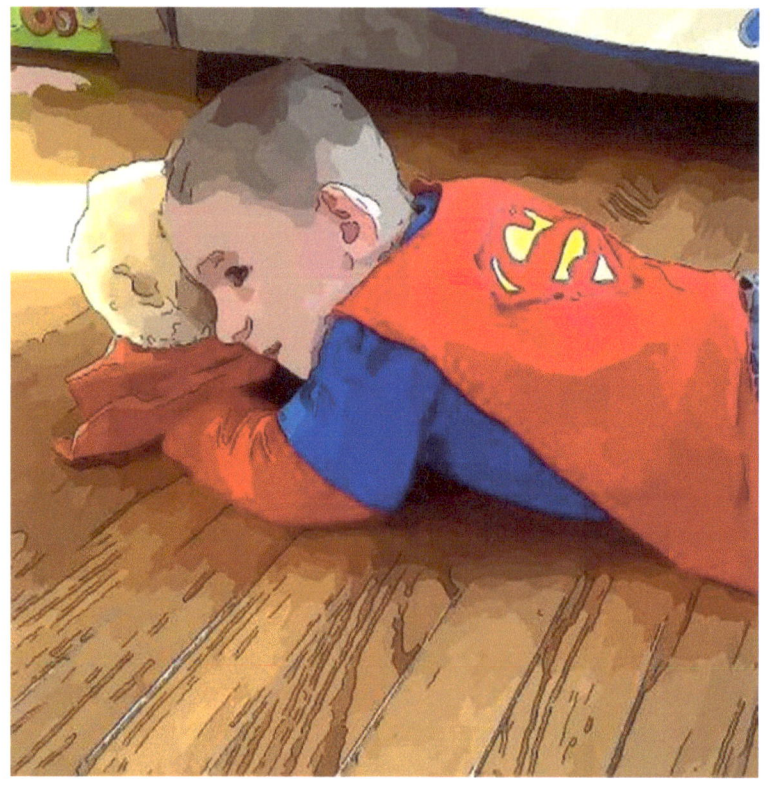

When life's challenges try to get in your way, Super Matthew
will save the day.

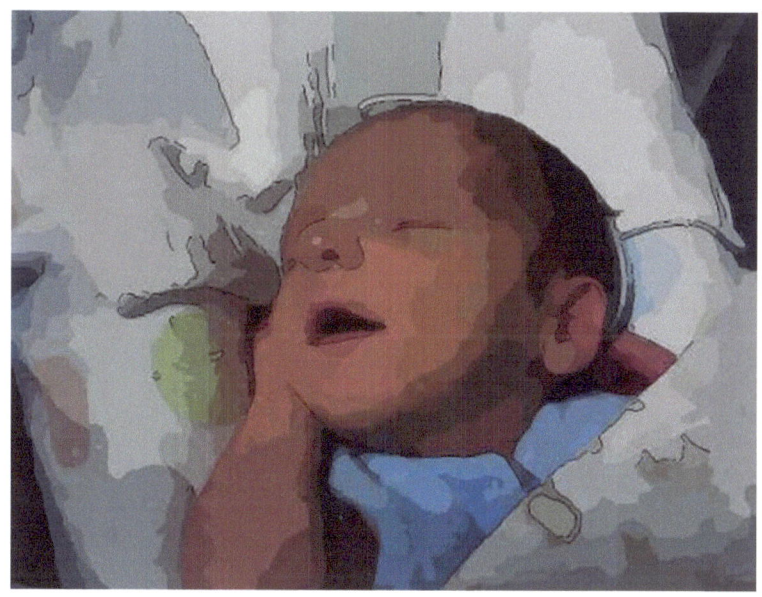

When Matthew was just a new-born boy, a tumor tried to steal his joy.

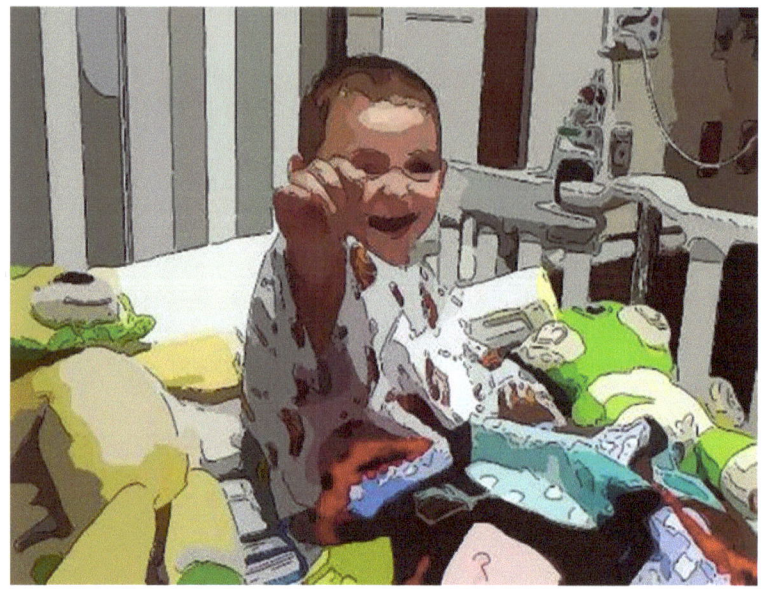

With his little hands and little feet, he knew that he could not be beat.

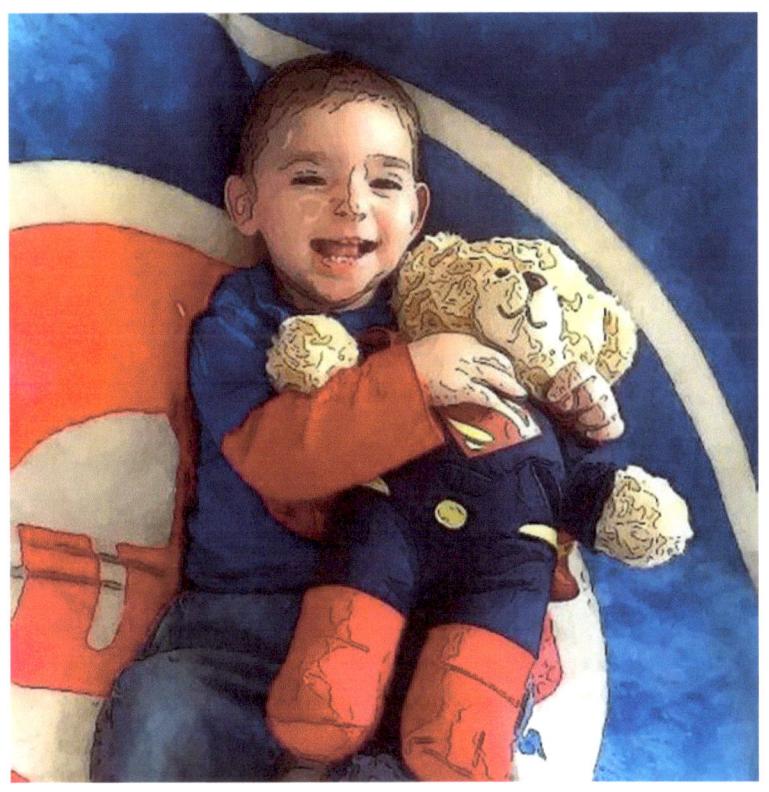

Those cancer cells were really mad that they couldn't keep Super Matthew sad.

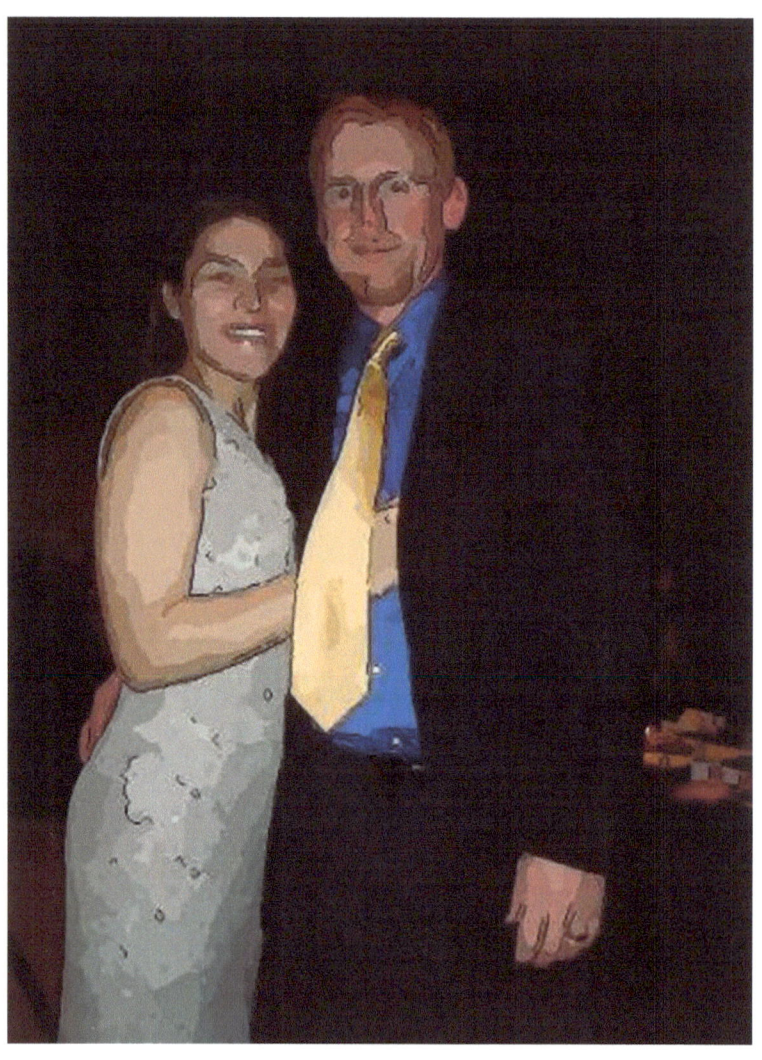

His mom and dad were super strong too, I'm sure that helped
Super Matthew get through.

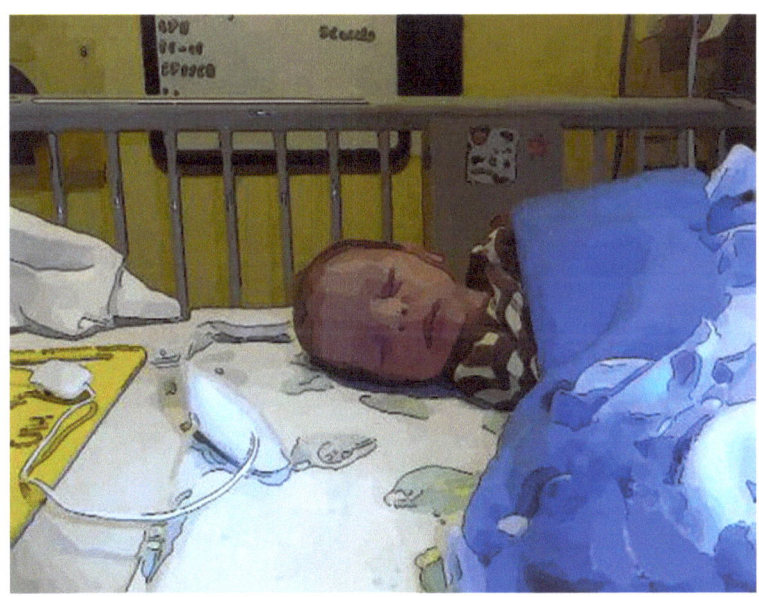

When Super Matthew went to sleep at night, he'd start to prepare for his fight.

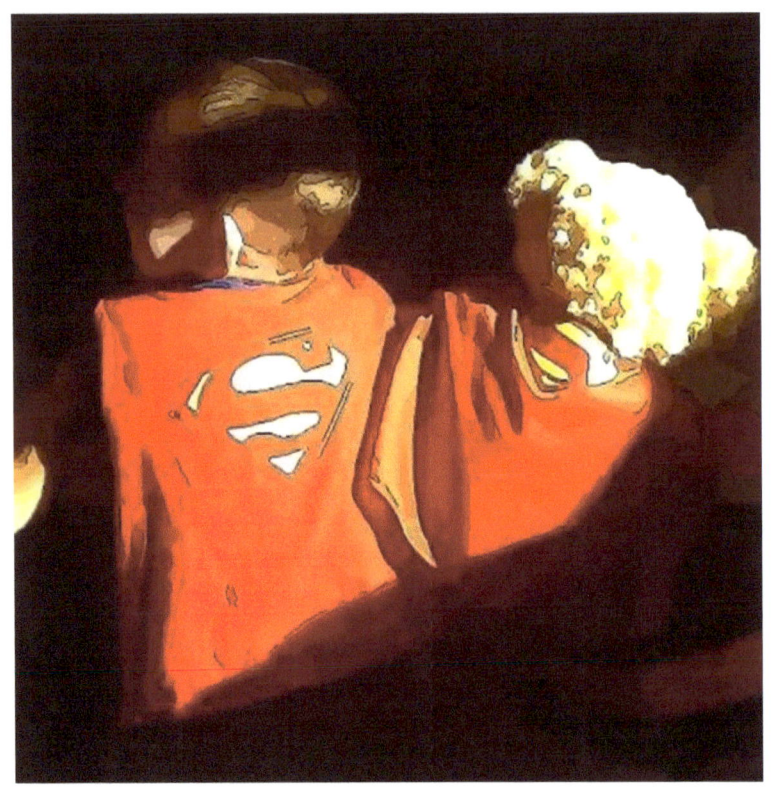

With his Super Teddy and cape in place, he knew what he
would have to face.

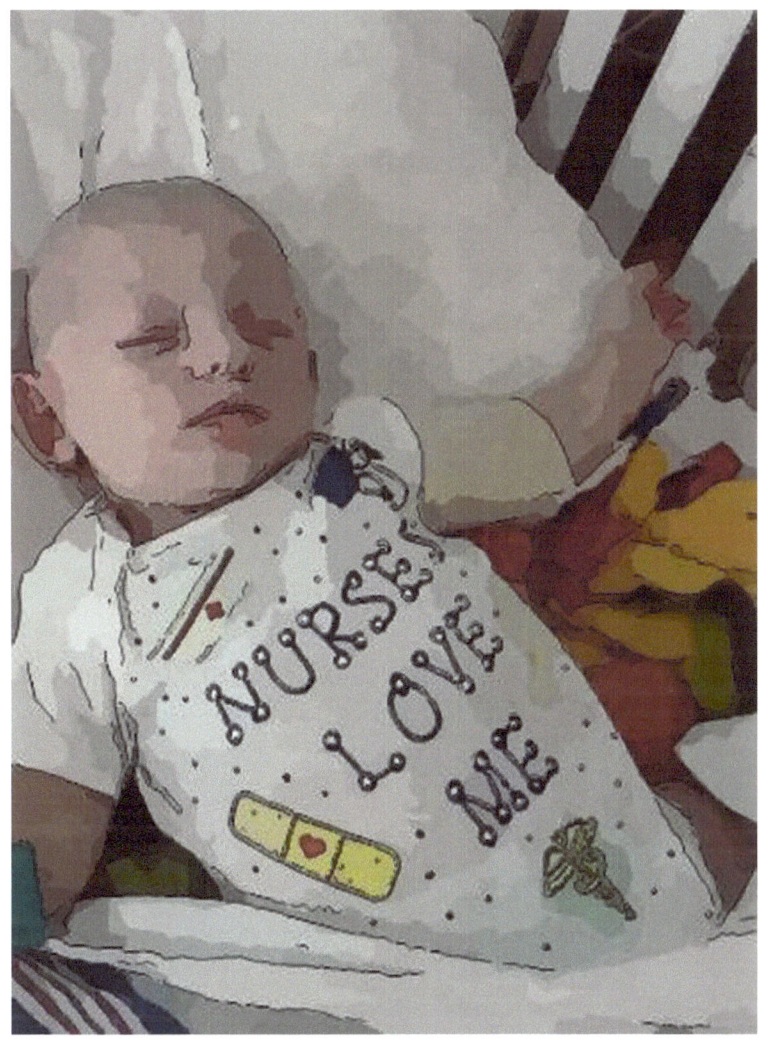

He'd close his eyes and go deep inside to find out where the bad cells hide,

Once he found them then he'd say. "Hey cancer cells you go away!"

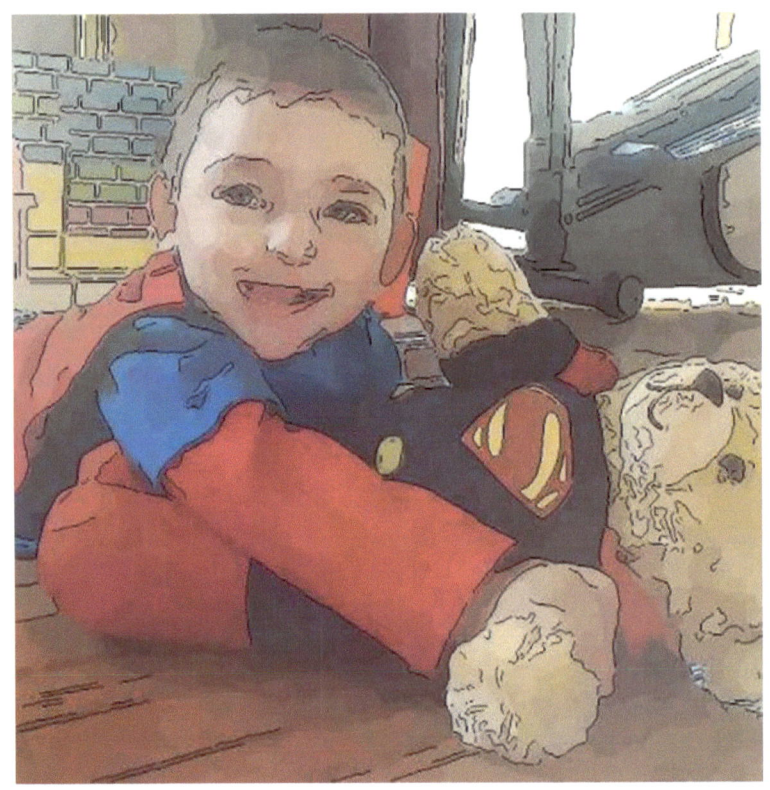

Some wouldn't listen and tried to stay, but with his super mind he pushed them away.

That tumor didn't have a chance once Super Matthew took his stance.

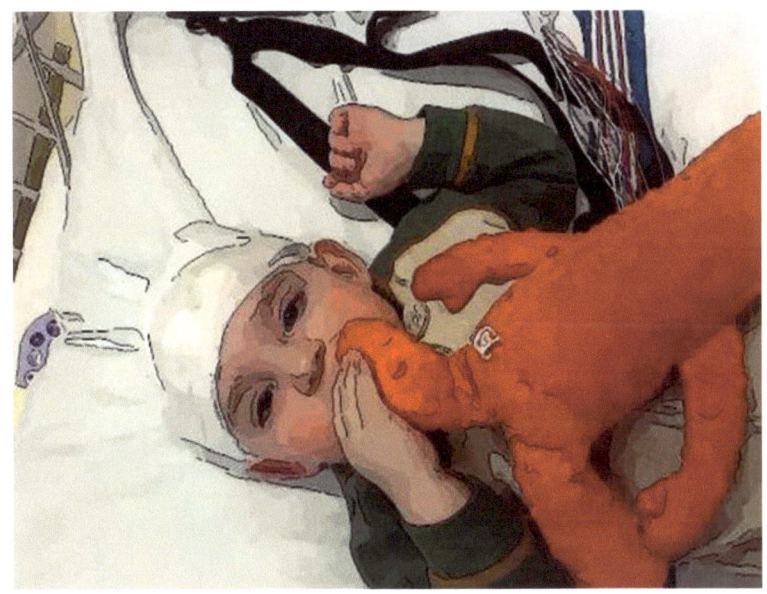

Once he opened his little eyes the doctors told him the big surprise.

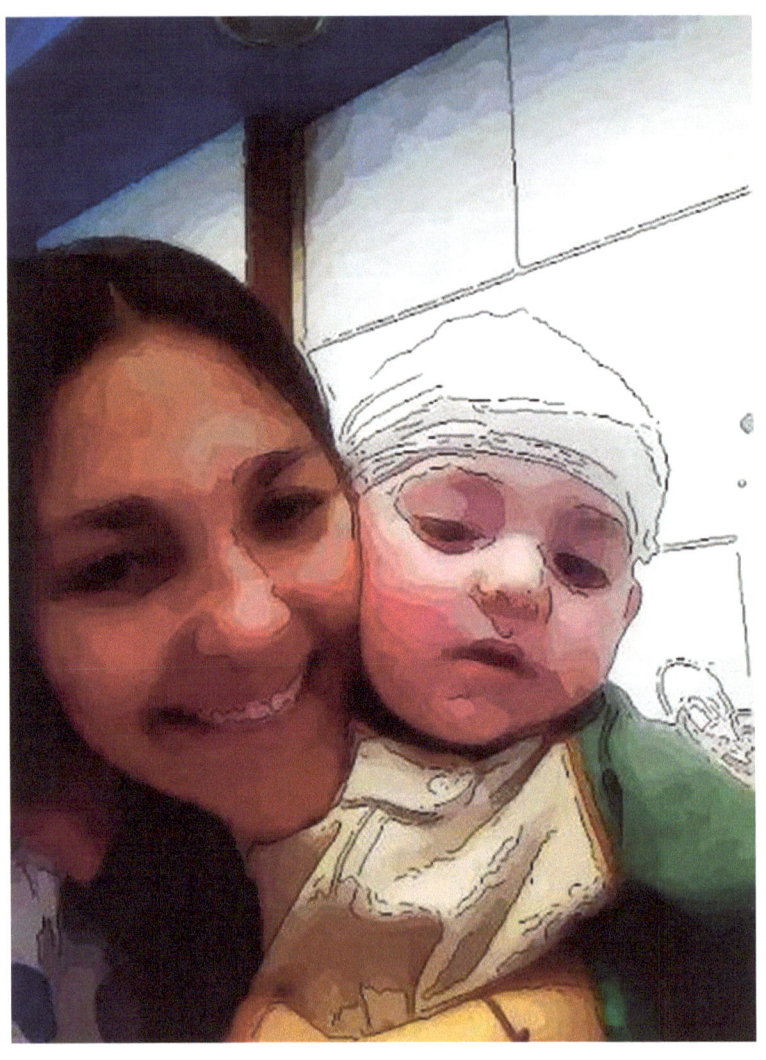

"The tumor is stable, no new growth was found"

Super Matthew's parents wanted to dance around.

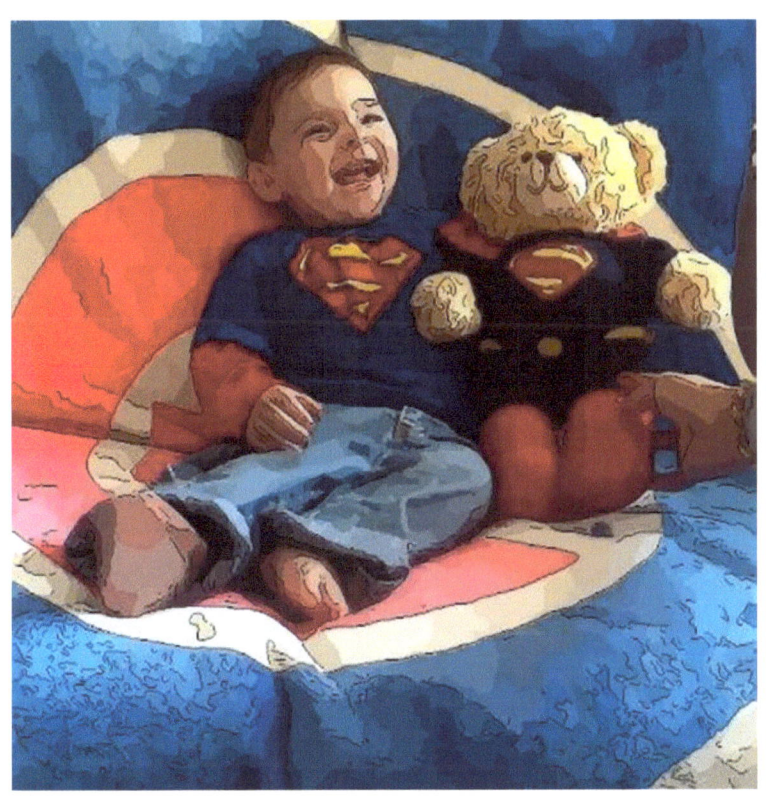

With a smile on his face from ear to ear,

Super Matthew never had any fear.

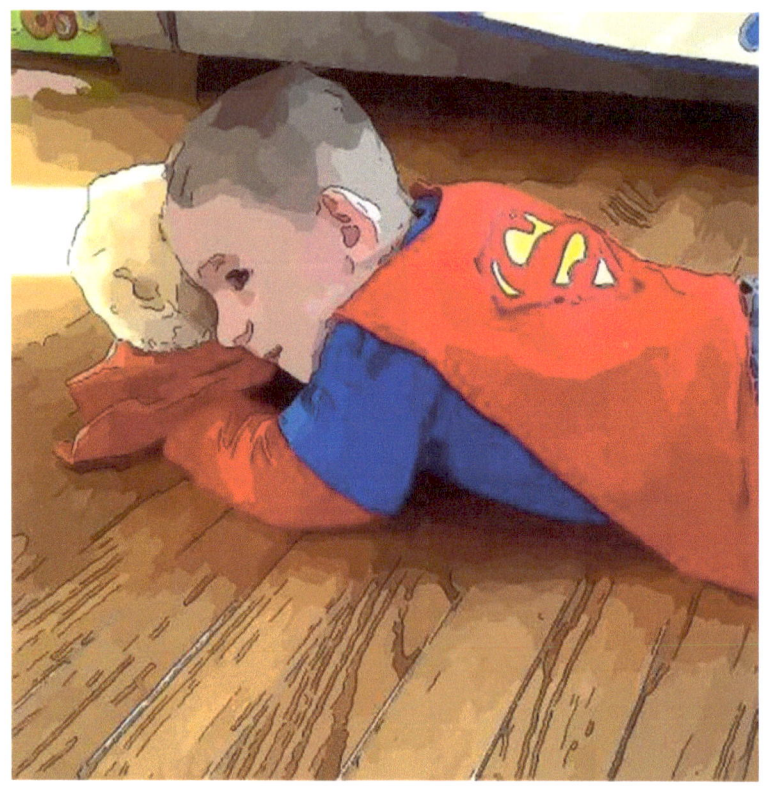

Everything would be okay because Super Matthew would save the day.

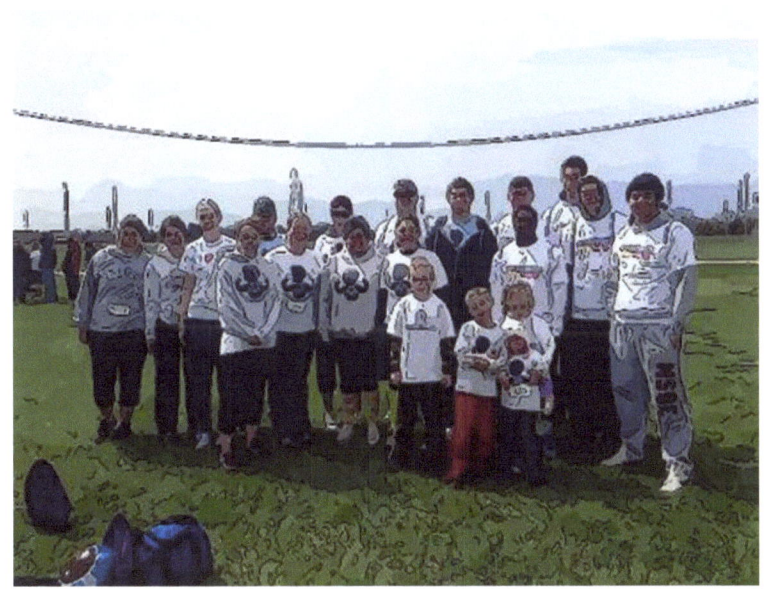

The Doctors and nurses and family helped too.

Special thanks to all those on team Super Matthew.

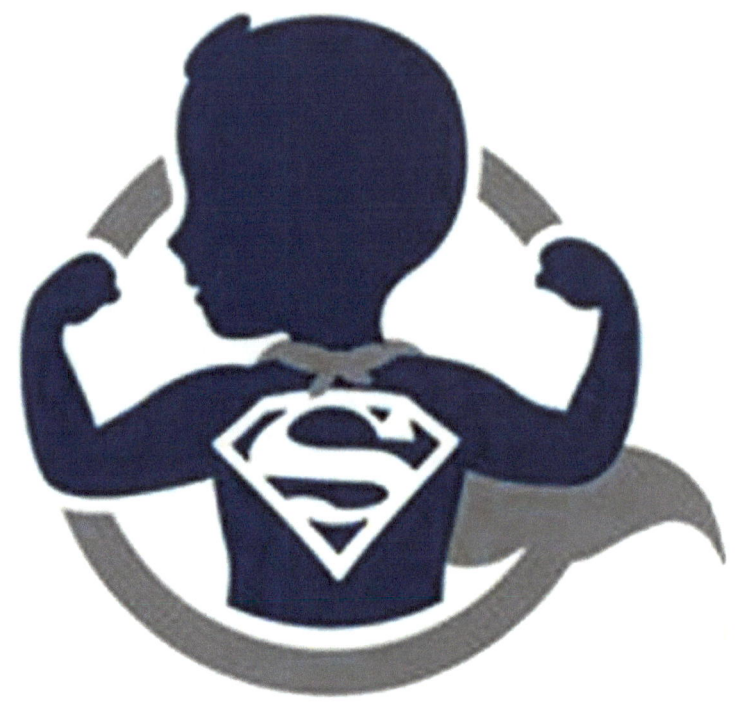

For those fighting life's challenges and need help making it through,

When you go to sleep at night think of Super Matthew.

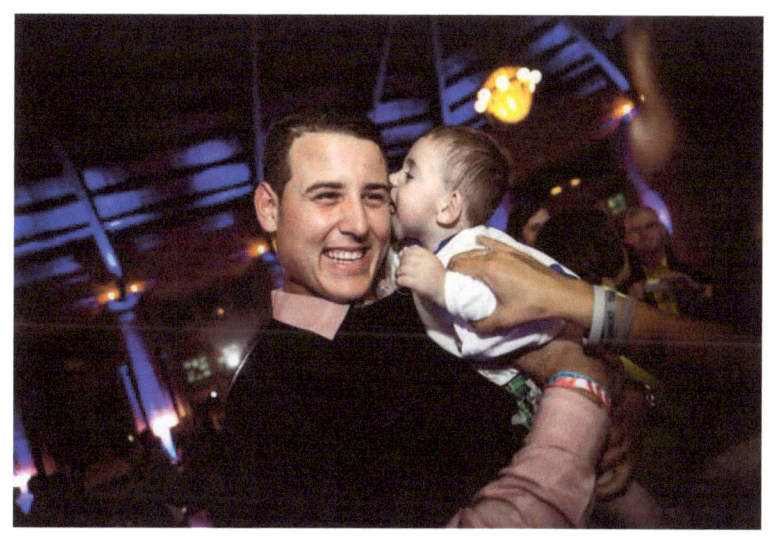

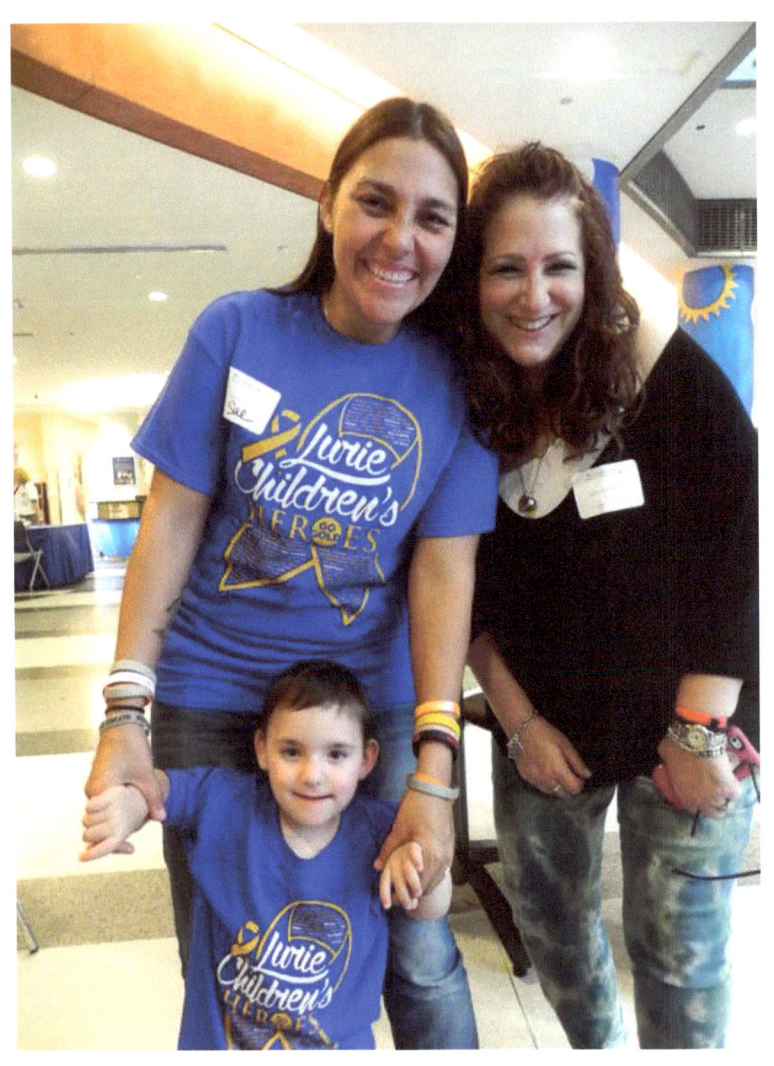

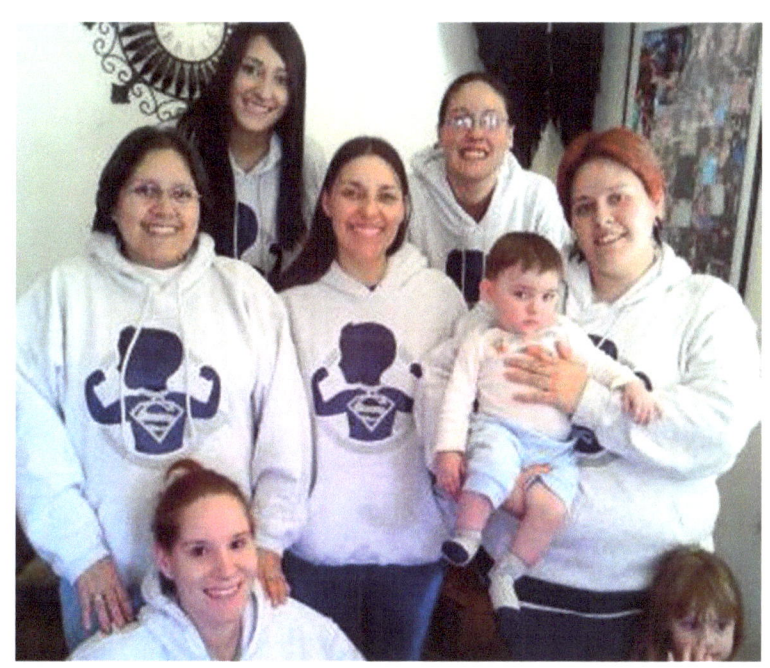

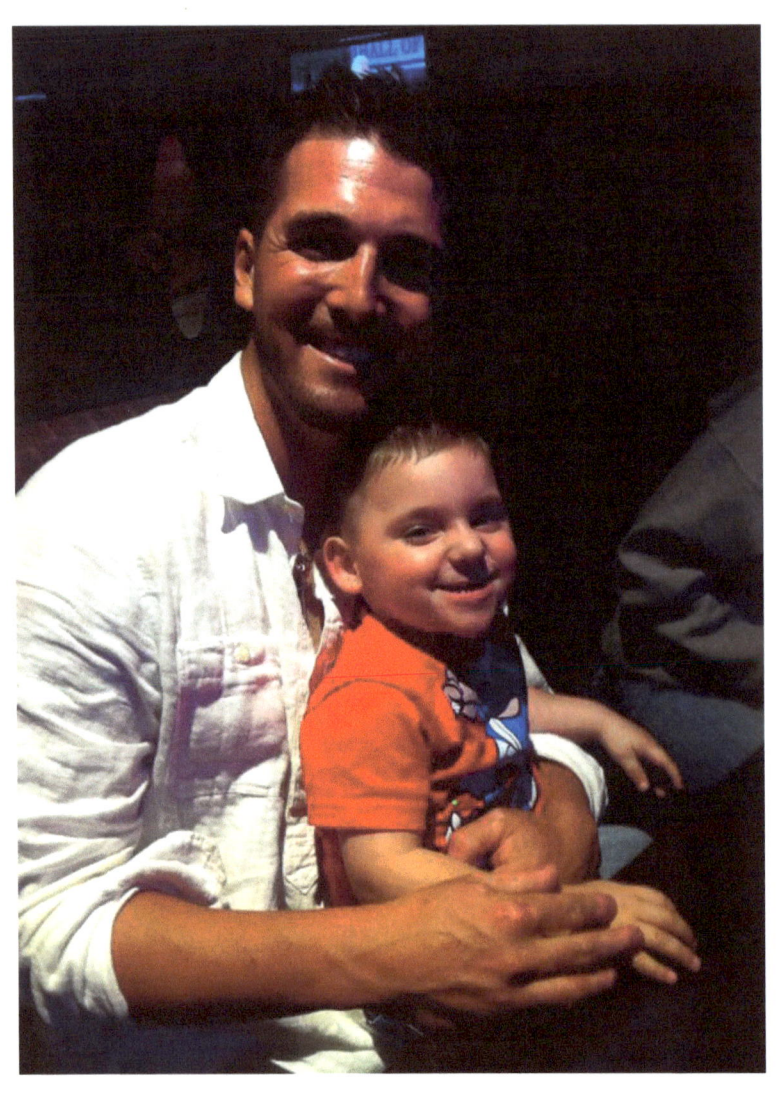

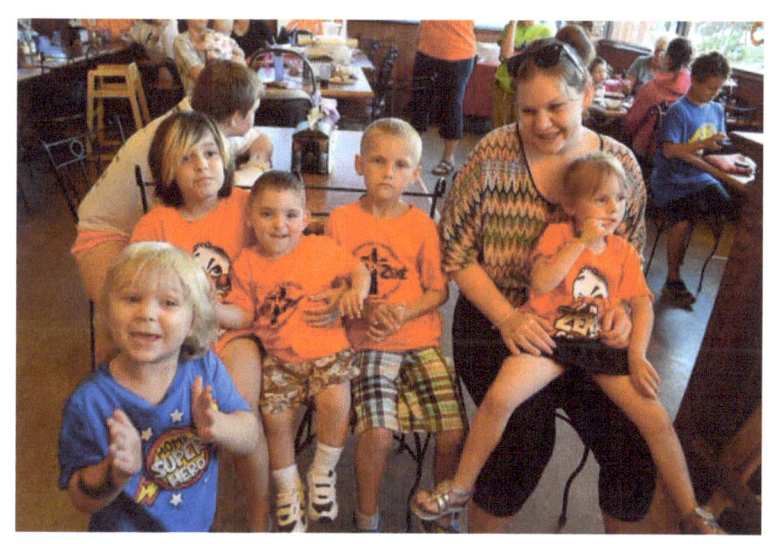

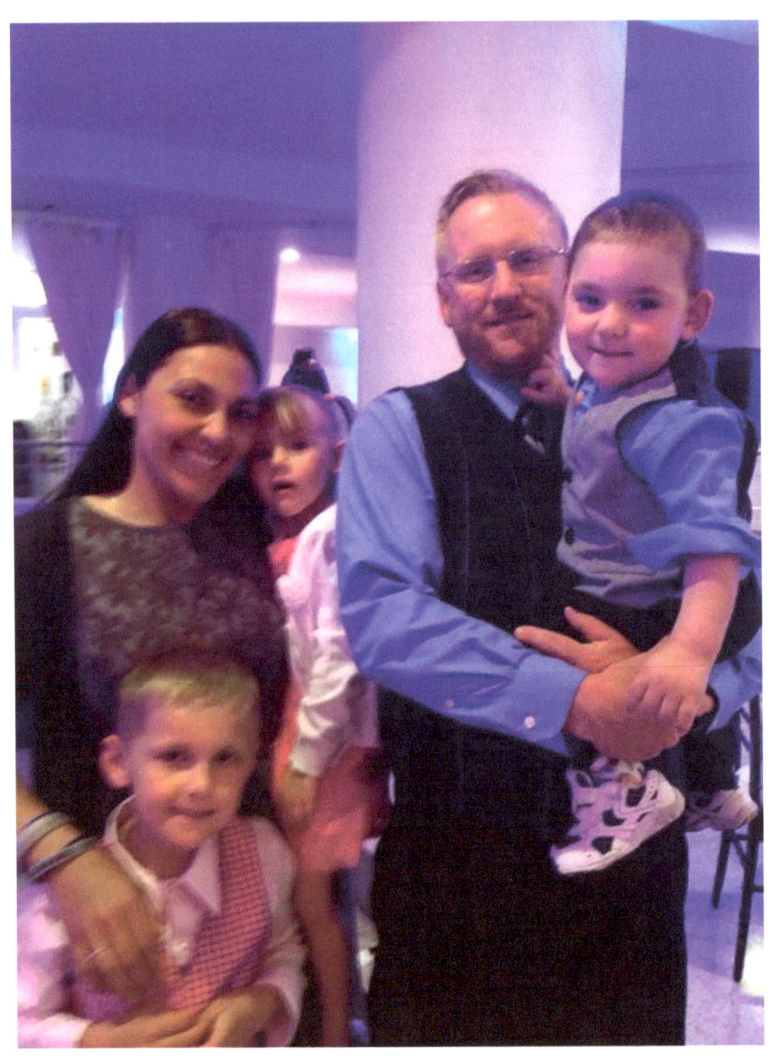

www.ingramcontent.com/pod-product-compliance
Lightning Source LLC
Chambersburg PA
CBHW041619180526
45159CB00002BC/928